DIVINE HEALTH AFFIRMATIONS AGAINST MALARIA

.....A Therapy that Works....

BY
IHEKE WILLIAMS

TABLE OF CONTENT

COPYRIGHT © 2019, IHEKE WILLIAMS

Unless otherwise indicated, all scripture quotations are taken from the King James Version of the Bible
A key for other Bible versions used;

NKJV	New King James Version
AMP	The Amplified Bible
TANT	The New Amplified Bible
TLB -	The Living Bible
CEV -	Contemporary English Version
NASB	New American Standard Version
GW -	God's Word version
ESV -	English Standard Version
NET -	New English Translation
ISV -	International Standard Version
NIV -	New International Version
MSG -	The Message Translation

DEDICATION

This Book is dedicated to Almighty God and to everyone in the world.

WHAT IS MALARIA?

Malaria is a mosquito-borne infectious disease affecting humans and other animals caused by single-celled microorganisms belonging to the plasmodium group.

Malaria causes symptoms that typically include fever, tiredness, vomiting and headaches. In severe cases it can cause yellow skin, seizures, coma or death. Symptoms usually begin ten to fifteen days after being bitten by an infected mosquito.

Source: Wikipedia

WHAT IS GOD'S SOLUTION

"...By His wounds ye have been healed.."- 1 Peter 2:24

JESUS has already healed you over 2000 years ago.

You have NO business with malaria.

You are Active and Strong forever because of the wound Jesus suffered on the cross for your sake.

For the next 31 days, you will affirm this blessing in your life and you will live free from malaria FOREVER.

<u>INSTRUCTION 1</u>

That if thou shalt confess with thy mouth the Lord Jesus, and shalt believe in thine heart that God hath raised him from the dead, thou shalt be saved. – Romans 10:9

There has to be a connection with what you say and what you have in your heart. We believe with our heart, this is the reason you have to meditate on the gospel with your heart, believe it and then affirm it.

For the affirmations to be effective, you will have to meditate on the scripture (1Peter 2:24) for 5 minutes, in your heart, and then affirm it.

INSTRUCTION 2

"For our light affliction, which is but for a moment, worketh for us a far more exceeding and eternal weight of glory;

While we look not at the things which are seen, but at the things which are not seen: for the things which are seen are temporal; but the things which are not seen are eternal. –
2 Corinthians 4:17-18

Don't look at the mirror or yourself during the duration of the affirmation. It affects the word in your heart when you keep seeing the sickness on your face.

Do not lie in bed all day. Get up and be active because Jesus has healed you. Do some house chores or something.

Follow these instructions and your affirmations will be more effective.

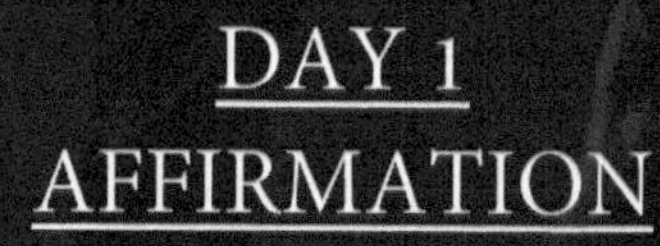

DAY 1
AFFIRMATION

Meditate on 1 Peter 2:24B in
your heart for 5 minutes
"..By His stripes ye have been
healed.."

Now Affirm the Blessing

"I HAVE BEEN HEALED THEREFORE, I AFFIRM THAT I DO NOT HAVE MALARIA INSIDE ME!"

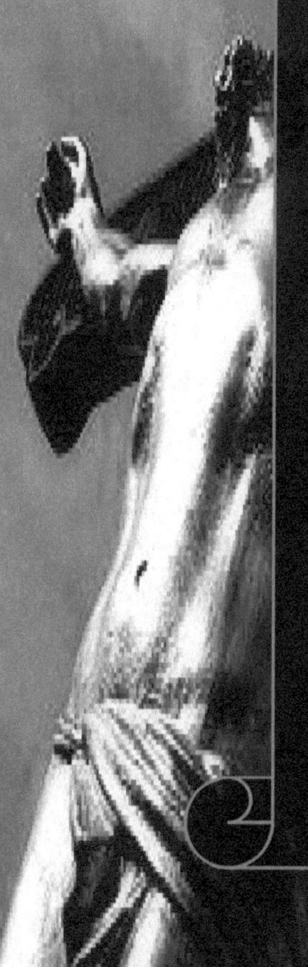

<u>DAY 2</u>
<u>AFFIRMATION</u>

Meditate on 1 Peter 2:24B in your heart for 5 minutes
"..By His stripes ye have been healed.."

Now Affirm the Blessing

"I HAVE BEEN HEALED THEREFORE, I AFFIRM THAT MY BODY IS ACTIVE AND STRONG FOREVER!"

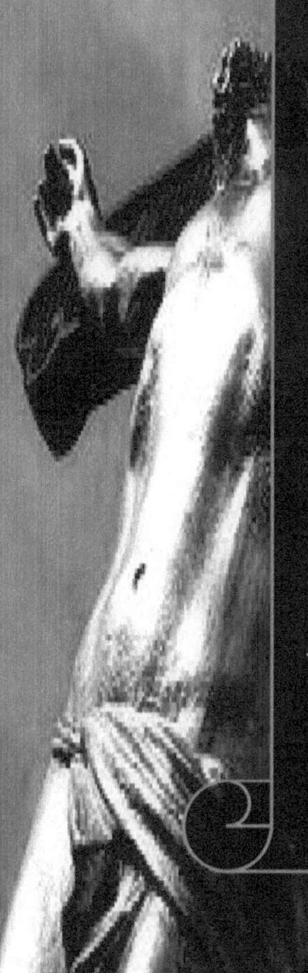
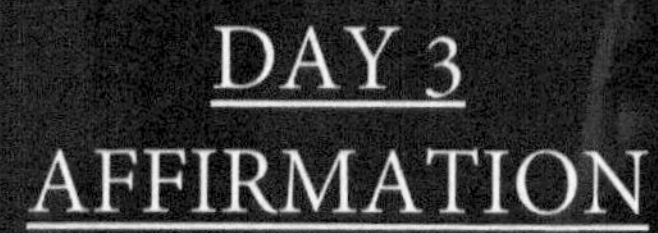

DAY 3
AFFIRMATION

Meditate on 1 Peter 2:24B in
your heart for 5 minutes
"..By His stripes ye have been
healed.."

Now Affirm the Blessing

"I HAVE BEEN
HEALED
THEREFORE, I
AFFIRM THAT I
DO NOT HAVE
MALARIA INSIDE
ME!"

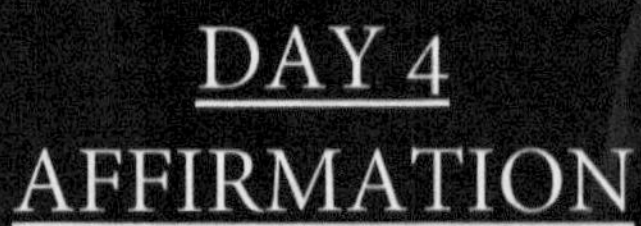

DAY 4
AFFIRMATION

Meditate on 1 Peter 2:24B in your
heart for 5 minutes
"..By His stripes ye have been
healed.."

Now Affirm the Blessing

"I HAVE BEEN
HEALED
THEREFORE, I
AFFIRM THAT MY
BODY IS ACTIVE
AND STRONG
FOREVER!"

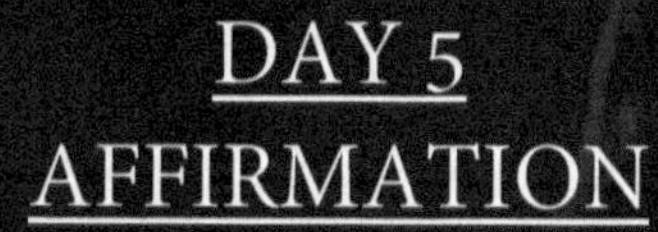
DAY 5
AFFIRMATION

Meditate on 1 Peter 2:24B in your heart for 5 minutes
"..By His stripes ye have been healed.."

Now Affirm the Blessing

"I HAVE BEEN HEALED THEREFORE, I AFFIRM THAT I DO NOT HAVE MALARIA INSIDE ME!"

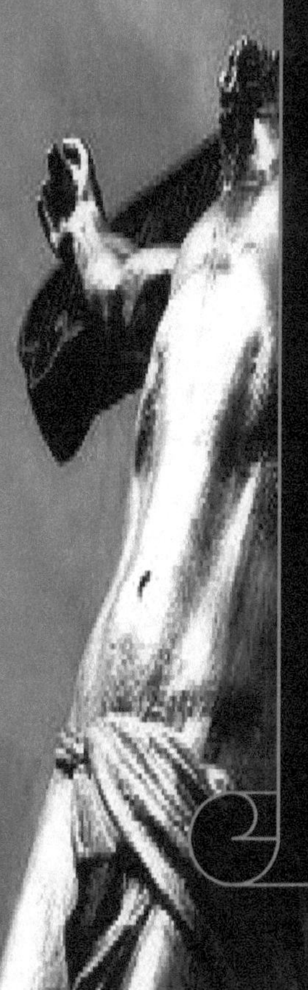

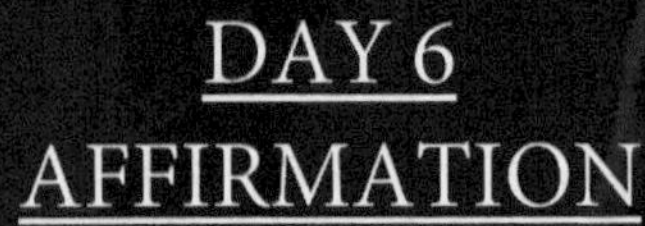

DAY 6
AFFIRMATION

Meditate on 1 Peter 2:24B in your heart for 5 minutes
"..By His stripes ye have been healed.."

Now Affirm the Blessing

"I HAVE BEEN HEALED THEREFORE, I AFFIRM THAT MY BODY IS ACTIVE AND STRONG FOREVER!"

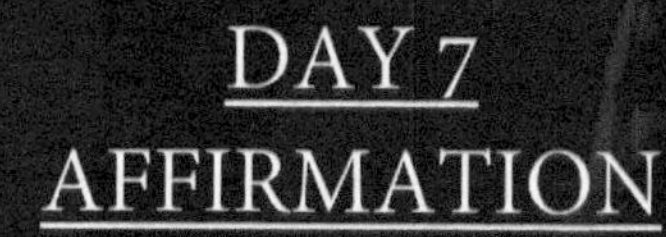

DAY 7
AFFIRMATION

Meditate on 1 Peter 2:24B in
your heart for 5 minutes
"..By His stripes ye have been
healed.."

Now Affirm the Blessing

"I HAVE BEEN HEALED THEREFORE, I AFFIRM THAT I DO NOT HAVE MALARIA INSIDE ME!"

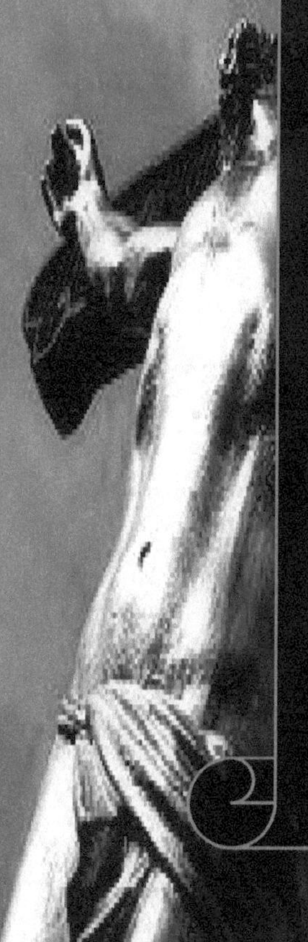

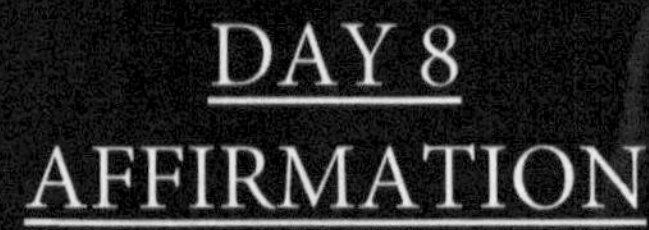

DAY 8
AFFIRMATION

Meditate on 1 Peter 2:24B in your
heart for 5 minutes
"..By His stripes ye have been
healed.."

Now Affirm the Blessing

"I HAVE BEEN HEALED THEREFORE, I AFFIRM THAT I AM ACTIVE AND STRONG FOREVER!"

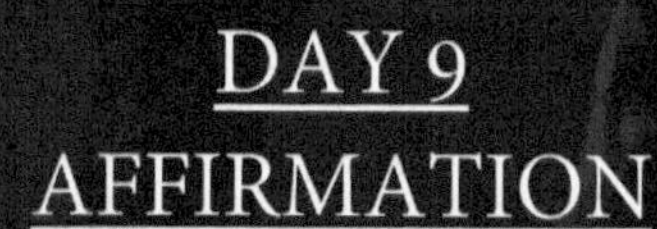

DAY 9
AFFIRMATION

Meditate on 1 Peter 2:24B in your heart for 5 minutes

"..By His stripes ye have been healed.."

Now Affirm the Blessing

"I HAVE BEEN HEALED THEREFORE, I AFFIRM THAT I DO NOT HAVE MALARIA INSIDE ME!"

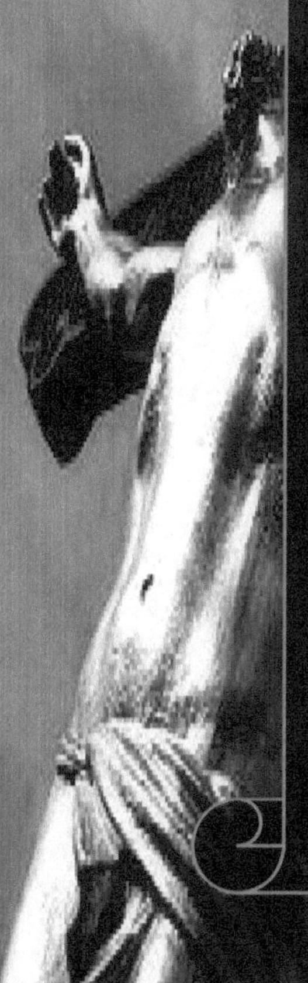

DAY 10
AFFIRMATION

Meditate on 1 Peter 2:24B in your
heart for 5 minutes
" ..By His stripes ye have been
healed.."

Now Affirm the Blessing

"I HAVE BEEN HEALED THEREFORE, I AFFIRM THAT I AM ACTIVE AND STRONG FOREVER!"

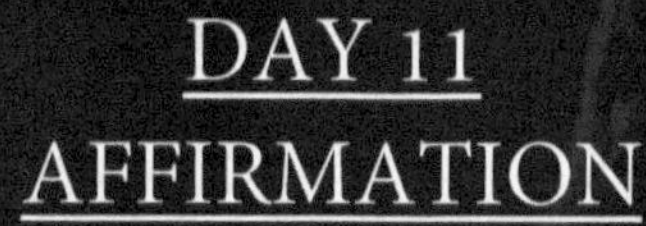

DAY 11
AFFIRMATION

Meditate on 1 Peter 2:24B in your heart for 5 minutes
"..By His stripes ye have been healed.."

Now Affirm the Blessing

"I HAVE BEEN HEALED THEREFORE, I AFFIRM THAT I DO NOT HAVE MALARIA INSIDE ME!"

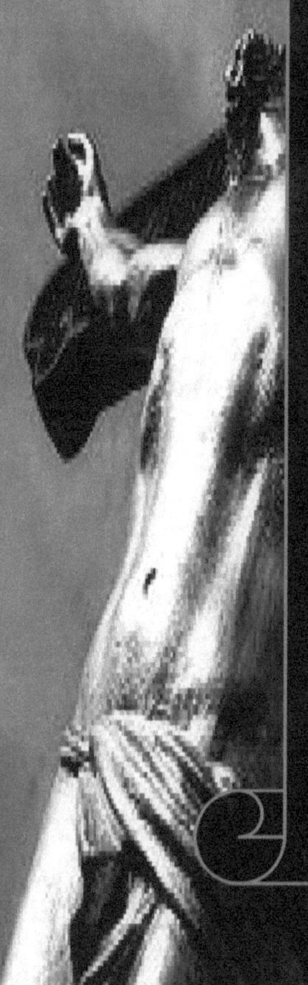

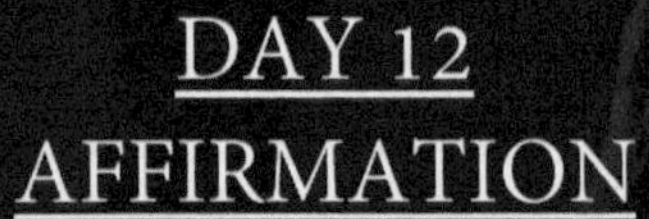

DAY 12
AFFIRMATION

Meditate on 1 Peter 2:24B in your
heart for 5 minutes
"..By His stripes ye have been
healed.."

Now Affirm the Blessing

"I HAVE BEEN HEALED THEREFORE, I AFFIRM THAT I AM ACTIVE AND STRONG FOREVER!"

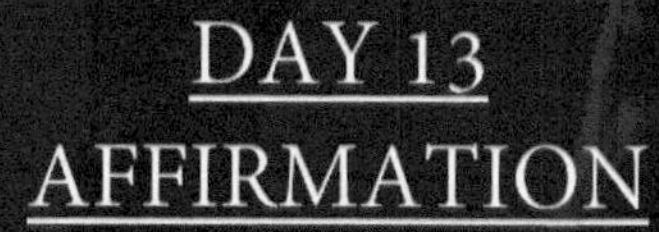

DAY 13
AFFIRMATION

Meditate on 1 Peter 2:24B in
your heart for 5 minutes
"..By His stripes ye have been
healed.."

Now Affirm the Blessing

"I HAVE BEEN HEALED THEREFORE, I AFFIRM THAT I DO NOT HAVE MALARIA INSIDE ME!"

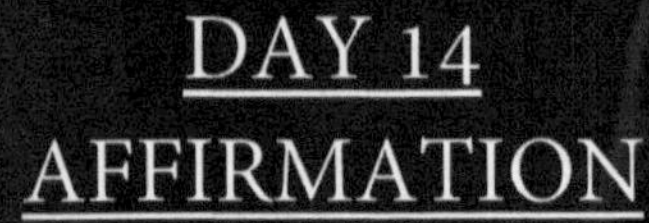

DAY 14
AFFIRMATION

Meditate on 1 Peter 2:24B in your heart for 5 minutes
"..By His stripes ye have been healed.."

Now Affirm the Blessing

"I HAVE BEEN HEALED THEREFORE, I AFFIRM THAT I AM ACTIVE AND STRONG FOREVER!"

DAY 15
AFFIRMATION

Meditate on 1 Peter 2:24B in your heart for 5 minutes
"..By His stripes ye have been healed.."

Now Affirm the Blessing

"I HAVE BEEN HEALED THEREFORE, I AFFIRM THAT I DO NOT HAVE MALARIA INSIDE ME!"

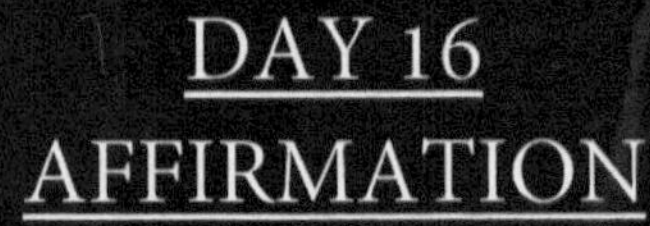

DAY 16
AFFIRMATION

Meditate on 1 Peter 2:24B in your
heart for 5 minutes
"..By His stripes ye have been
healed.."

Now Affirm the Blessing

"I HAVE BEEN
HEALED
THEREFORE, I
AFFIRM THAT I AM
ACTIVE AND
STRONG
FOREVER!"

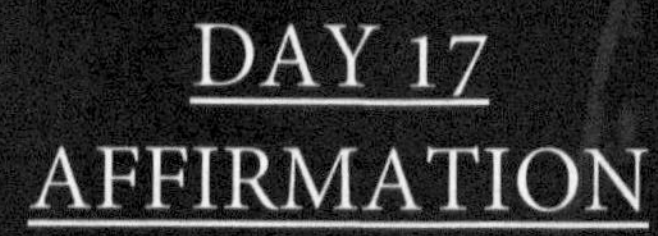
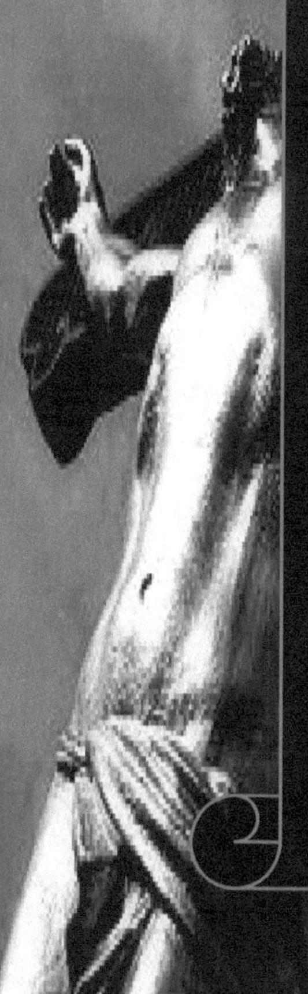

DAY 17
AFFIRMATION

Meditate on 1 Peter 2:24B in your heart for 5 minutes
"..By His stripes ye have been healed.."

Now Affirm the Blessing

"I HAVE BEEN HEALED THEREFORE, I AFFIRM THAT I DO NOT HAVE MALARIA INSIDE ME!"

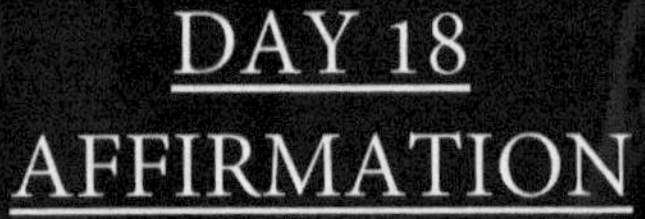

DAY 18
AFFIRMATION

Meditate on 1 Peter 2:24B in your heart for 5 minutes
"..By His stripes ye have been healed.."

Now Affirm the Blessing

"I HAVE BEEN HEALED THEREFORE, I AFFIRM THAT I AM ACTIVE AND STRONG FOREVER!"

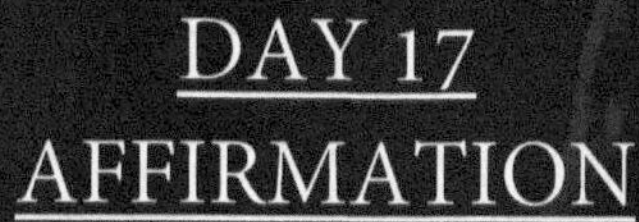

DAY 17
AFFIRMATION

Meditate on 1 Peter 2:24B in your heart for 5 minutes
"..By His stripes ye have been healed.."

Now Affirm the Blessing

"I HAVE BEEN HEALED THEREFORE, I AFFIRM THAT I DO NOT HAVE MALARIA INSIDE ME!"

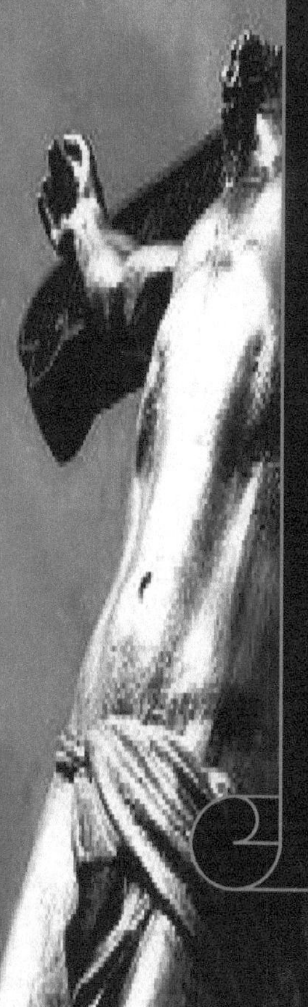

DAY 18
AFFIRMATION

Meditate on 1 Peter 2:24B in your heart for 5 minutes
"..By His stripes ye have been healed.."

Now Affirm the Blessing

"I HAVE BEEN HEALED THEREFORE, I AFFIRM THAT I AM ACTIVE AND STRONG FOREVER!"

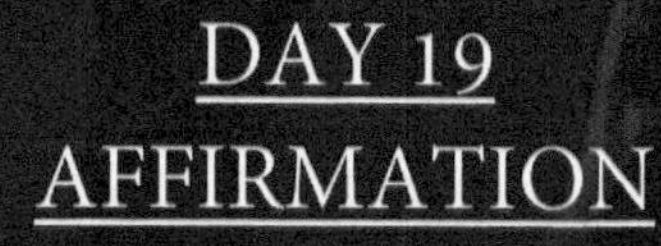

DAY 19
AFFIRMATION

Meditate on 1 Peter 2:24B in
your heart for 5 minutes
"..By His stripes ye have been
healed.."

Now Affirm the Blessing

"I HAVE BEEN HEALED THEREFORE, I AFFIRM THAT I DO NOT HAVE MALARIA INSIDE ME!"

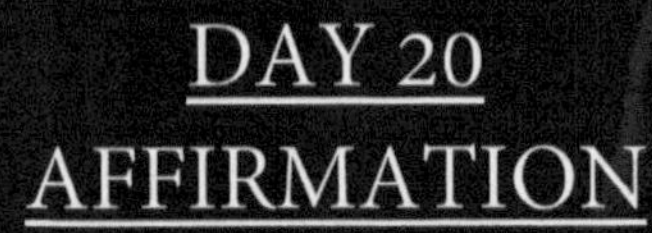

DAY 20
AFFIRMATION

Meditate on 1 Peter 2:24B in your heart for 5 minutes
"..By His stripes ye have been healed.."

Now Affirm the Blessing

"I HAVE BEEN HEALED THEREFORE, I AFFIRM THAT I AM ACTIVE AND STRONG FOREVER!"

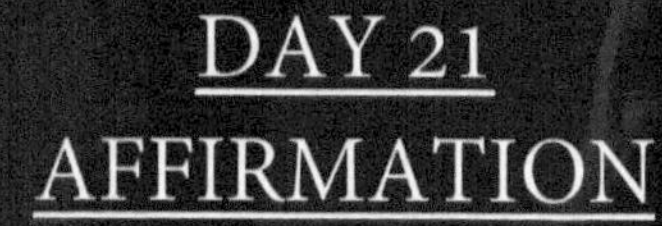

DAY 21
AFFIRMATION

Meditate on 1 Peter 2:24B in your heart for 5 minutes
"..By His stripes ye have been healed.."

Now Affirm the Blessing

"I HAVE BEEN HEALED THEREFORE, I AFFIRM THAT I DO NOT HAVE MALARIA INSIDE ME!"

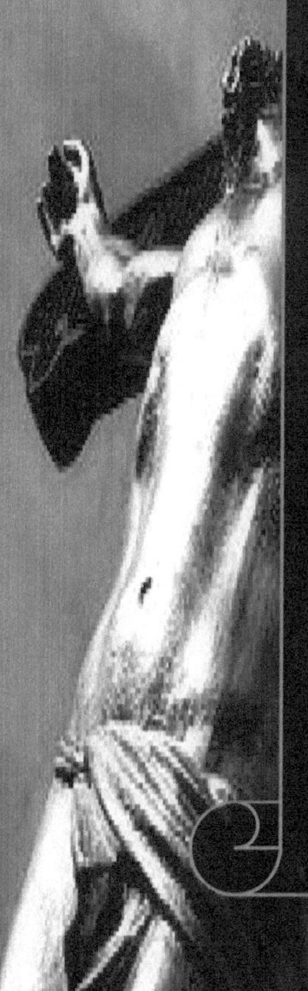

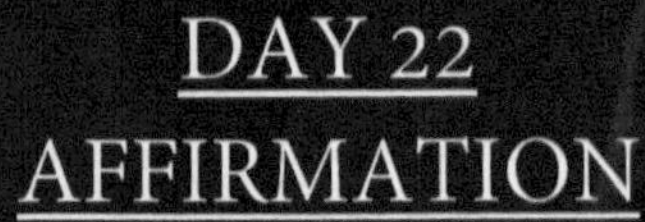

DAY 22
AFFIRMATION

Meditate on 1 Peter 2:24B in your
heart for 5 minutes
"..By His stripes ye have been
healed.."

Now Affirm the Blessing

"I HAVE BEEN HEALED THEREFORE, I AFFIRM THAT I AM ACTIVE AND STRONG FOREVER!"

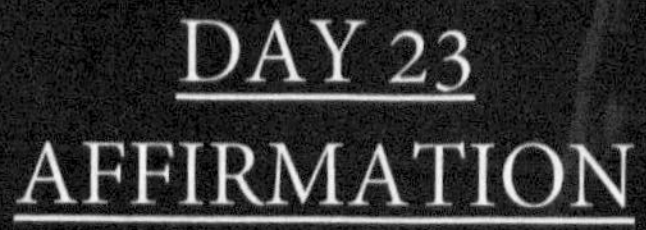
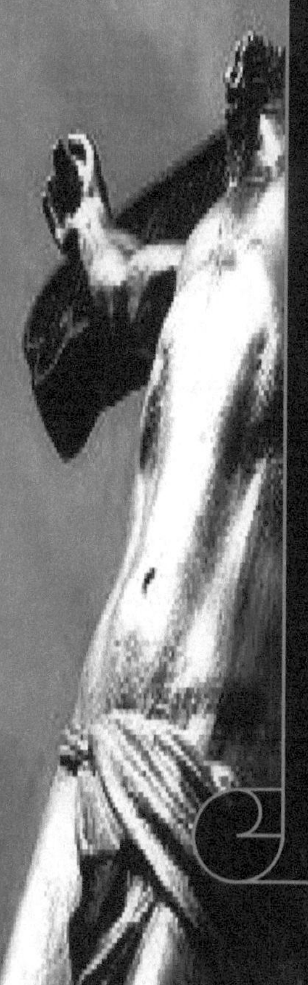

DAY 23
AFFIRMATION

Meditate on 1 Peter 2:24B in your heart for 5 minutes
"..By His stripes ye have been healed.."

Now Affirm the Blessing

"I HAVE BEEN HEALED THEREFORE, I AFFIRM THAT I DO NOT HAVE MALARIA INSIDE ME!"

DAY 24
AFFIRMATION

Meditate on 1 Peter 2:24B in your
heart for 5 minutes
"..By His stripes ye have been
healed.."

Now Affirm the Blessing

"I HAVE BEEN HEALED THEREFORE, I AFFIRM THAT I AM ACTIVE AND STRONG FOREVER!"

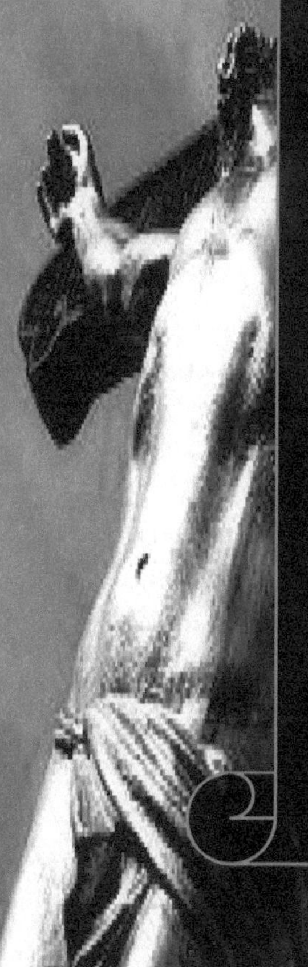

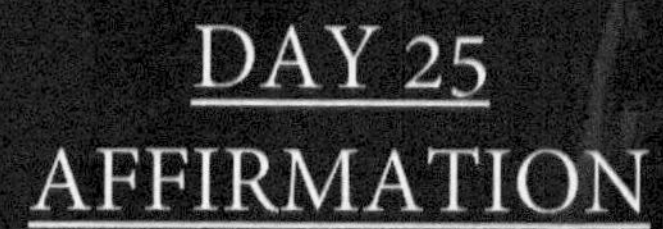

DAY 25
AFFIRMATION

Meditate on 1 Peter 2:24B in
your heart for 5 minutes
" ..By His stripes ye have been
healed.."

Now Affirm the Blessing

"I HAVE BEEN HEALED THEREFORE, I AFFIRM THAT I DO NOT HAVE MALARIA INSIDE ME!"

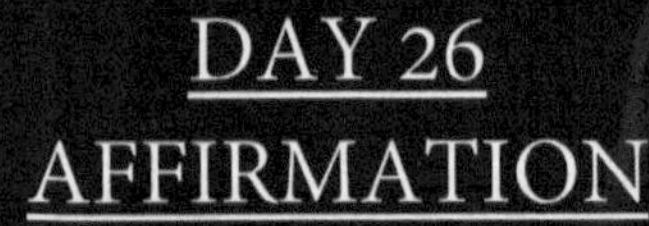

DAY 26
AFFIRMATION

Meditate on 1 Peter 2:24B in your
heart for 5 minutes
"..By His stripes ye have been
healed.."

Now Affirm the Blessing

"I HAVE BEEN
HEALED
THEREFORE, I
AFFIRM THAT I AM
ACTIVE AND
STRONG
FOREVER!"

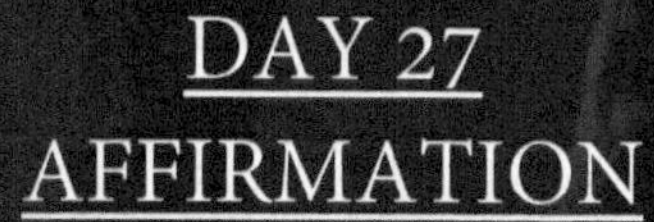

DAY 27
AFFIRMATION

Meditate on 1 Peter 2:24B in
your heart for 5 minutes
"..By His stripes ye have been
healed.."

Now Affirm the Blessing

"I HAVE BEEN HEALED THEREFORE, I AFFIRM THAT I DO NOT HAVE MALARIA INSIDE ME!"

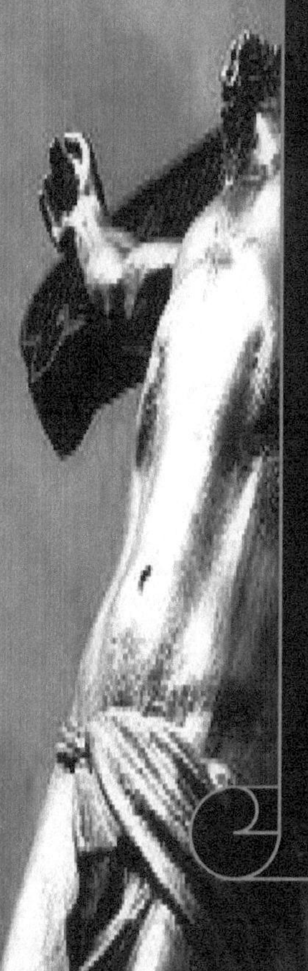

DAY 28
AFFIRMATION

Meditate on 1 Peter 2:24B in your heart for 5 minutes
" ..By His stripes ye have been healed.."

Now Affirm the Blessing

"I HAVE BEEN HEALED THEREFORE, I AFFIRM THAT MY BODY IS ACTIVE AND STRONG FOREVER!"

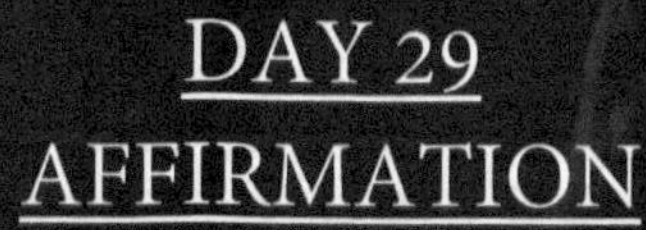

DAY 29
AFFIRMATION

Meditate on 1 Peter 2:24B in
your heart for 5 minutes
"..By His stripes ye have been
healed.."

Now Affirm the Blessing

"I HAVE BEEN HEALED THEREFORE, I AFFIRM THAT I DO NOT HAVE MALARIA INSIDE ME!"

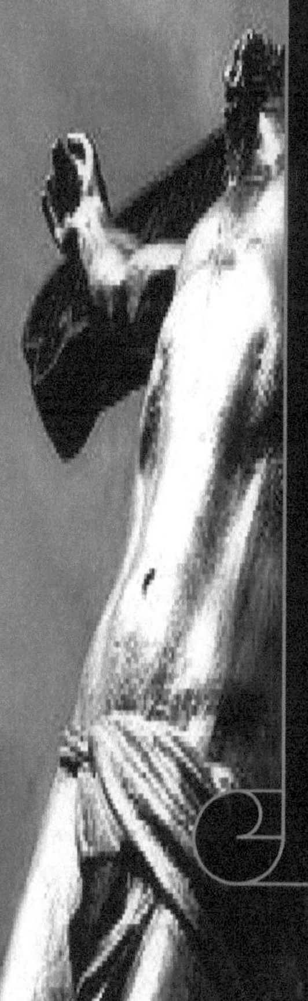

DAY 30
AFFIRMATION

Meditate on 1 Peter 2:24B in your
heart for 5 minutes
"..By His stripes ye have been
healed.."

Now Affirm the Blessing

"I HAVE BEEN HEALED THEREFORE, I AFFIRM THAT MY BODY IS ACTIVE AND STRONG FOREVER!"

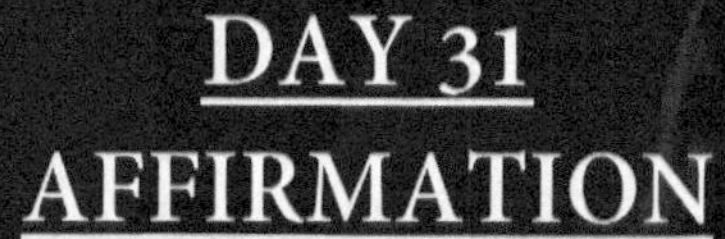

DAY 31
AFFIRMATION

Meditate on 1 Peter 2:24B in your heart for 5 minutes
"..By His stripes ye have been healed.."

Now Affirm the Blessing

"I HAVE BEEN HEALED THEREFORE, I AFFIRM THAT I AM ACTIVE AND STRONG FOREVER!"

SUMMARY

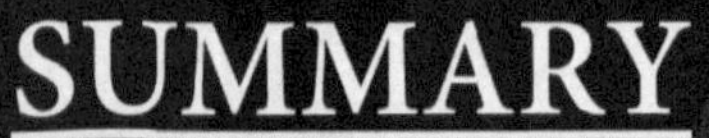

"..By His stripes ye have been healed.."- 1 Peter 2:24

Malaria does not exist in you. JESUS has healed you already.

Rejoice and live in Divine Health all the days of your life.

YOU ARE ACTIVE AND STRONG FOREVER!!!

PRAYER FOR SALVATION

We believe that you have been blessed and that you want to receive eternal life that God has made available to everyone who believes in his love and his grace which He expressed lavishly through His Son Jesus Christ.

"For God so loved the world, that He gave his only begotten Son, that whosoever believeth in him should not perish, but have everlasting life." - John 3:16

Say this prayer to God and believe it with your heart

"Father, I believe that you gave me your only Son to die for my sin. I believe you raised Him from the dead. I declare that your son, Jesus Christ is the Lord of my life. I receive eternal life and I receive the Holy Spirit. I am saved forever.in Jesus name. I am so Happy that today and forever, I am your child. Amen ".

Congratulations, you are now a child of God Halleluyah!! — John 1:12

<u>OTHER INFORMATION</u>

Please share your testimonies via the following handles;

ihekewilliams@gmail.com
+2348061530541

Other Books written by the author includes
Dad, Pray for your Daughter
Mum, Pray for your Daughter
Mum, pray for your Son
Don't stop the flow of the Blessing
Daddy's Prayers
Mummy's Prayers
Divine Health Affirmation Against Cancer
Divine Health Affirmations Against Migraine Headaches
Divine Health Affirmation Against kidney Failure
Divine Health Affirmation Against Heart Failure
Divine Health Affirmations Series

ABOUT THE AUTHOR

Iheke Williams is a firm follower and disciple of the Lord Jesus Christ. He is a passionate minister of the grace of our Lord and savior Jesus Christ and has brought the reality of the divine life of Christ into the lives of so many.

Iheke Williams has a calling to communicate the gospel of Christ with simplicity and to show the world how to activate the eternal life of God that is in us already which includes Divine health, Divine righteousness, Divine security and Divine prosperity.

As you read this book and other books written by Iheke Williams you will literally begin to function and manifest the life of God that is already inside you to the glory of God the Father who is the author of all grace and mercy. Amen!

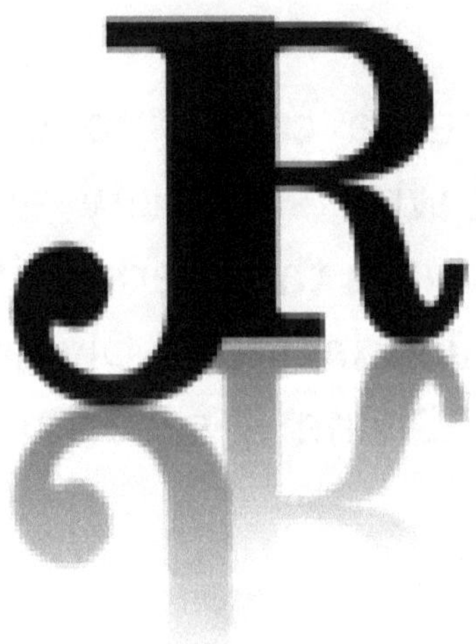